Amanda Duling

Amanda Duling, M.S.
Founder, One Gear Short of Normal™

First Edition · Version 1.0 · March 2026

Published by **One Gear Short of Normal™**

Disclaimer

This guide is for informational purposes only and is not intended to diagnose, treat, or provide medical advice. Always consult your licensed healthcare provider before making changes to your training, nutrition, equipment, or product use. Amanda Duling is not a licensed medical professional. Participation is voluntary and at your own risk.

How This Guide Is Designed

This guide is written for endurance coaches and athletes who treat pain, hygiene, and recovery as performance variables — not rites of passage. The structure is intentional: clear hierarchy, minimal visual noise, and rules that prioritize usability under fatigue, time pressure, and real-world training conditions. Humor is used sparingly to address topics that are often ignored, not to undermine rigor. This is a reference document, not a manifesto, and it is meant to be revisited, shared, and applied.

TABLE OF CONTENTS

QUICK START: READ THIS FIRST IF YOU'RE SHORT ON TIME

If you only read three sections, start here:

- The Four-Factor Problem: Friction, Heat, Pressure, Moisture
- When Pain Isn't Normal
- The Recovery Protocol: Clean → Soothe → Restore

QUICK REFERENCE TABLE

Symptom	Likely Cause	First Action
Chafing or raw skin	Friction combined with trapped moisture	Check chamois fit, reduce seams, apply a barrier cream
Burning or stinging sensation	Product irritation or pH imbalance	Stop product use, rinse area gently, allow skin to calm
Numbness	Excess pressure on the perineum	Stop riding, reassess saddle width, tilt, and position
Recurrent saddle sores	Skin breakdown with bacterial involvement	Follow the recovery protocol; consider diluted Hibiclens if needed
Swelling or tenderness	Heat and prolonged pressure	Reduce ride duration, improve airflow, reassess saddle setup
Persistent moisture	Poor airflow or non-breathable fabrics	Switch to moisture-wicking kit, change out of gear promptly
Slow healing skin	Low estrogen or compromised skin barrier	Prioritize recovery time; avoid riding on damaged skin
Pain that worsens over time	Mechanical issue or fit mismatch	Stop riding and address saddle fit before continuing

WHY THIS GUIDE EXISTS

"Pain isn't grit. It's data."

That's...a lot of butt stuff.

My aunt said that the first time she walked into my bathroom. She wasn't wrong. To the untrained eye, it looks like a pharmaceutical crime scene: balms, creams, tubs labeled things like "Euro style" that could either heal your skin or strip paint.

To an endurance cyclist, it's survival gear.

Here's the problem: most cycling guidance around saddle pain, chafing, and numbness was never written for women. Less than 15% of saddle-pressure studies even include female anatomy. The result is a culture where discomfort is normalized, silence is expected, and real injuries are brushed off as "part of riding."

This guide exists to break that pattern.

We're going to talk about anatomy, friction, sweat, nerves, hormones, and recovery — clearly, scientifically, and without euphemisms. Because comfort isn't weakness. It's how you stay on the bike.

WHO THIS GUIDE IS FOR

This guide is for you if:

- You ride longer than 60 minutes and saddle pain lingers
- You've been told discomfort is "just part of cycling"
- You are post-bariatric, perimenopausal, menopausal, or hormonally shifting
- You care about longevity, not just grit

WHAT'S ACTUALLY HAPPENING DOWN THERE

> ## If you don't know what's rubbing, you can't fix it.

Let's stop saying "down there" and start being accurate.

Vulva: External genitalia — labia, clitoris, vaginal opening. Delicate tissue, not built for constant friction.
Perineum: The strip of tissue between the vaginal opening and anus. Your saddle's favorite target.
Urethral opening: Easily irritated by heat, pressure, forward saddle tilt, and migrating creams.

Your saddle should support your **sit bones** — the ischial tuberosities. Everything else is soft tissue, and soft tissue is not meant to bear load for hours.

When saddle width, tilt, or position is wrong, pressure shifts forward. That leads to friction, swelling, micro-tears, numbness, and infection risk. This isn't about toughness. It's biomechanics.

THE FOUR-FACTOR PROBLEM: FRICTION, HEAT, PRESSURE, MOISTURE

"It's not sweat — it's physics."

Every pedal stroke creates shear forces between your skin and chamois. Friction generates heat. Heat increases sweat. Sweat breaks down the skin barrier and feeds bacteria and fungi.

Once moisture is trapped, skin enters **maceration** — the over-hydrated, fragile state that makes tissue prone to breakdown.

This creates a feedback loop:

- Friction raises heat
- Heat increases sweat
- Sweat fuels microbes
- Microbes damage skin
- Damaged skin increases friction

Female anatomy makes this worse. More folds. Less airflow. More moisture retention. Hormonal shifts — especially reduced estrogen — thin skin and slow healing.

This is why chafing isn't random. It's predictable.

And solvable.

BUILD YOUR BUTT ARSENAL (MATCH THE TOOL TO THE RIDE)

**Your lube should match
your ride — not your mood.**

There is no single "best" chamois cream. There is only the one that fits your skin, sweat rate, hormones, and conditions.

The Three Product Categories

Silicone-based
Best for: long, hot, wet rides
Pros: water-resistant, long-lasting
Cons: can clog pores if not washed off well

Water-based
Best for: short to medium rides, sensitive skin
Pros: breathable, easy cleanup
Cons: breaks down fast with sweat

Zinc or lanolin balms
Best for: recovery, irritated skin
Pros: healing, protective
Cons: heavy, can stain fabric

How to Choose

- **Heavy sweater?** Silicone or hybrid
- **Sensitive skin?** Fragrance-free, pH-balanced
- **Low estrogen weeks?** Barrier-based zinc creams

Rule of thumb: *If it stings, it's not courage — it's chemistry.*
Test new products on short rides. Wash thoroughly post-ride.
Think toolbox, not shrine.

CHAMOIS & SKIN PROTECTION MATRIX					
Ride Length	**Heat**	**Sweat Rate**	**Skin State**	**Recommended Product Category**	**Why This Works**
Short (<90 min)	Cool	Low	Normal	Water-based	Breathable, low buildup, easy cleanup
Short (<90 min)	Hot	High	Normal	Hybrid (water + light silicone)	Adds durability without heavy occlusion
Medium (90–180 min)	Cool	Low	Sensitive	Water-based (fragrance-free)	Minimizes irritation, maintains airflow
Medium (90–180 min)	Hot	High	Normal	Silicone-based	Resists sweat breakdown and shear forces
Medium (90–180 min)	Hot	High	Sensitive	Hybrid or light silicone	Balances protection with skin tolerance
Long (3+ hrs)	Cool	Low	Normal	Silicone-based	Long-lasting friction protection

Long (3+ hrs)	Hot	High	Normal	Silicone-based	Maximum durability in wet, high-shear conditions
Long (3+ hrs)	Any	Any	Low-estrogen weeks	Zinc or barrier-based	Protects fragile skin, reduces micro-tearing
Recovery / Irritated Skin	N/A	N/A	Raw or inflamed	Zinc or lanolin balm	Healing, protective, antimicrobial support

Quick Interpretation Rules

More heat   +   More sweat   = More barrier

Longer rides   = Durability over breathability

Sensitive or low-estrogen skin = Protection over performance

- If it stings, burns, or worsens after the ride — stop using it
- If friction persists, reassess saddle fit and position before adding more product

WHEN PAIN ISN'T NORMAL

"Numbness is not a badge of honor."

The perineum contains critical nerves and blood vessels. Prolonged compression can restrict blood flow and irritate the pudendal nerve.

Stop and reassess if you experience:

- Numbness lasting more than 10–15 minutes post-ride
- Burning or electric sensations
- Tingling down the inner thigh
- Swelling or deep ache that doesn't resolve overnight

These are neurological warning signs — not training adaptations.

Modern saddles, proper fit, and small positional changes can dramatically reduce risk. If symptoms persist, consult a pelvic floor physical therapist, sports medicine physician, or urogynecologist familiar with cycling.

Pain is data. Listen to it.

HORMONES, BARIATRIC SURGERY, AND SKIN REALITY

> ## Your body didn't fail.
> ## The playbook changed.

Estrogen supports skin elasticity, moisture, and repair. When levels drop — menopause, certain medications — skin becomes thinner and more fragile.

Post-bariatric athletes face additional changes:

- Altered sweat chemistry
- pH shifts
- Skin folds that trap moisture
- Micronutrient deficiencies affecting healing

This requires adaptation, not shame.

Practical care:

- Gentle, pH-balanced cleansers
- Thorough drying (especially folds)
- Ceramide-rich moisturizers
- Zinc or antifungal protection where needed
- Monitoring zinc, iron, and vitamin A with a clinician

You're training in different biology. Adjust accordingly.

THE RECOVERY PROTOCOL: CLEAN → SOOTHE → RESTORE

"Recovery isn't optional. It's the next ride's foundation."

CLEAN

- Shower immediately post-ride
- Warm water, mild cleanser
- No scrubbing
- Diluted Hibiclens 1–2×/week if infection-prone

SOOTHE

- Zinc-based or healing balm
- Skip menthol and fragrance
- Rest if skin is raw or swollen

RESTORE

- Respect pain lasting >24–48 hours
- Cold compresses or sitz baths for swelling
- Hydration + protein, zinc, vitamin A
- Replace worn-out chamois

Stop riding if you have:
persistent numbness, weeping sores, deep swelling, or sharp pain when sitting.

You wouldn't ignore a stress fracture. Don't ignore your perineum.

WHAT THIS ALL ADDS UP TO

Here's the truth no one told us:

- Comfort is not optional
- Silence doesn't equal toughness
- Longevity beats grit

You've earned your seat. Take care of the skin, nerves, and tissue that keep you there.

Clean. Soothe. Restore.
And refuse to normalize pain.

HOW THIS GUIDE WAS BUILT
(Credibility & Methodology)

This guide wasn't written from vibes, forums, or "what worked for me once."

It was built at the intersection of **peer-reviewed research, real-world endurance experience, and bodies that sports science routinely ignores.**

1. Evidence-Informed, Not Evidence-Blind

All scientific claims referenced in this guide are grounded in:

- Peer-reviewed journal articles
- Systematic reviews
- Sports medicine, dermatology, and biomechanics research

Topics supported by research include:

- Saddle pressure distribution and nerve compression
- Female-specific cycling anatomy and vascular effects
- Friction, heat, sweat, and skin barrier breakdown
- Hormonal influences on skin resilience and healing
- Post-bariatric physiological changes affecting skin and infection risk

Full citations are provided in the **References** section.

This guide does not present original research.
It translates existing research into plain language and practical application.

2. Real-World Athlete Translation

Research alone doesn't tell you:

- How skin behaves after 4 hours in heat and grit
- What happens when estrogen drops mid-training block
- Why certain "popular" products fail in high-sweat conditions
- How silence and normalization delay treatment and cause injury

This guide incorporates:

- Endurance cycling experience across long gravel and road rides
- Post-bariatric skin and sweat adaptation
- Menopause-related skin changes
- Trial-and-error product testing across conditions

The goal isn't perfection — **it's longevity.**

3. Clear Boundaries (Important)

This guide:

- Does **not** replace medical care
- Does **not** diagnose or treat conditions
- Does **not** recommend ignoring symptoms

It does:

- Help readers recognize warning signs
- Encourage appropriate escalation to professionals
- Provide prevention-focused, low-risk strategies

Comfort is framed as **injury prevention**, not indulgence.

4. Why These Topics Matter

Less than 15% of saddle-pressure studies include women.
Post-bariatric athletes are rarely addressed at all.
Menopause is treated like an afterthought in endurance sports.

This guide exists because:

- Pain has been mislabeled as toughness
- Silence has been confused with resilience
- Too many athletes quit not because they're weak — but because no one gave them usable information

5. Versioning & Updates

This is Version 1.0

Future updates may:

- Refine language
- Add new references
- Clarify protocols as research evolves

Buyers will receive updated versions when available.

Note: This guide is a living document. Future versions may refine language, add references, or clarify protocols as research evolves.

REFERENCE ALIGNMENT STATEMENT

All in-text scientific concepts referenced in this guide correspond directly to sources listed in the **References** section, including but not limited to:

- Saddle pressure, nerve compression, and vascular compression
  (Baranowski et al.; Bini & Hume; Schrader et al.; Bressel & Larson)
- Female genital anatomy, sensation, and cycling impact
  (Guess et al.; Kingsberg & Krychman)
- Friction, heat, sweat, and skin microclimate
  (Kottner et al.; Wilke et al.; Sommer et al.)
- Hormonal influences on skin integrity
  (Farage & Maibach; Lephart; Søndergaard & Nordin)
- Post-bariatric skin changes and infection risk
  (Hirsch et al.; Sarwer et al.)

No claims extend beyond the scope of cited evidence or clearly framed lived experience.

ABOUT THE AUTHOR

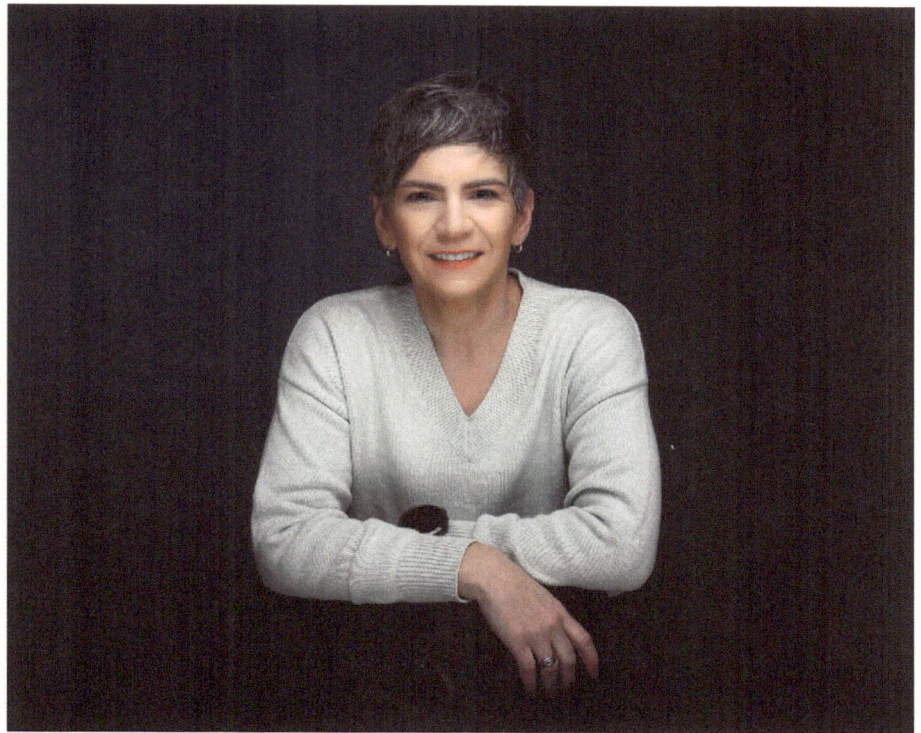

Amanda Duling is an endurance cyclist, post-bariatric athlete, and the writer behind *One Gear Short of Normal*™. She blends lived experience, evidence-based research, and dark humor to talk about the things athletes are told to endure quietly — and shouldn't.

REFERENCES

Baranowski, A. P., Anderson, K. E., & Brinsden, M. (2000). Pudendal nerve entrapment: An uncommon source of chronic perineal pain. British Journal of Urology International, 85(3), 313–318.

Bertuccio, M., et al. (2020). Influence of environmental conditions on cycling performance and comfort. European Journal of Applied Physiology, 120(2), 415–428. https://doi.org/10.1007/s00421-019-04277-9

Bini, R. R., & Hume, P. A. (2020). Gender differences in bicycle saddle pressure: A review. Sports Biomechanics, 19(3), 263–278.

Bini, R. R., Hume, P. A., & Croft, J. L. (2020). Effects of bicycle saddle on pelvic and perineal pressure in female cyclists: A systematic review. Journal of Science and Cycling, 9(1), 3–12.

Bini, R. R., Hume, P. A., & Croft, J. L. (2011). Effects of bicycle saddle height on knee injury risk and comfort. Sports Medicine, 41(6), 463–476.

Bressel, E., & Larson, B. J. (2003). Bicycle seat designs and their effect on perineal pressure. Medicine & Science in Sports & Exercise, 35(6), 1029–1033.

Draelos, Z. D. (2012). The effect of menopause on the skin and options for treatment. Clinics in Dermatology, 30(5), 595–601.

Farage, M. A., & Maibach, H. I. (2006). Influence of the menstrual cycle on the female skin. Contact Dermatitis, 54(4), 213–221.

Gehring, W., Matzke, D., & Hensel, E. (2008). Influence of saddle pressure distribution on genital numbness and saddle sores in female cyclists. Journal of Sports Science & Medicine, 7(3), 375–381.

Gemery, J. M., Nangia, A. K., Mamourian, A. C., & Reid, S. K. (2007). Digital three-dimensional modeling of the perineum and bicycle seats: Implications for perineal compression. Urology, 70(5), 910–915.

Guess, M. K., Connell, K. A., Schrader, S. M., Reutman, S. R., Wang, A., LaJoie, A. S., & Toennis, C. A. (2006). Genital sensation and sexual function in women bicyclists and runners: Are your genitals at risk? Journal of Sexual Medicine, 3(6), 1018–1027. https://doi.org/10.1111/j.1743-6109.2006.00298.x

Guess, M. K., Connell, K. A., Schrader, S., Reutman, S., Wang, A., LaJoie, A. S., & Toennis, C. (2010). Genital sensation and sexual function in women bicyclists and runners: Are your feet safer than your seat? Journal of Sexual Medicine, 7(5), 2139–2147.

Hirsch, A., et al. (2018). Skin changes after bariatric surgery: Review of the literature and management recommendations. Obesity Surgery, 28(12), 3896–3907.

Kingsberg, S. A., & Krychman, M. L. (2015). Resistance to estrogen therapy for vulvovaginal atrophy: Barriers, beliefs, and misperceptions. Journal of Sexual Medicine, 12(12), 2491–2497.

Kottner, J., et al. (2018). The role of skin microclimate in pressure injury development: A review. Journal of Tissue Viability, 27(2), 77–83. https://doi.org/10.1016/j.jtv.2018.02.001

Lephart, E. D. (2018). Skin aging and menopause: Implications for treatment. Dermato-Endocrinology, 10(1), e1442165. https://doi.org/10.1080/19381980.2018.1442165

Sarwer, D. B., et al. (2008). Changes in body image and quality of life following bariatric surgery. Obesity Surgery, 18(9), 1154–1159.

Schober, J. M., Lenschow, B. W., & Feustel, P. J. (2021). Effects of saddle design on female perineal anatomy and pressure distribution. Clinical Journal of Sport Medicine, 31(1), 47–53.

Schrader, S. M., Breitenstein, M. J., & Lowe, B. D. (2002). Cutting off the nose to save the penis. Journal of Sexual Medicine, 1(1), 33–40.

Sommer, F., König, D., Graft, C., Klotz, T., Engelmann, U., & Schmitz, H. (2001). Impaired blood flow and the risk of genital numbness in cyclists. Journal of Urology, 166(3), 1028–1031.

Søndergaard, M., & Nordin, J. M. (2020). Hormonal influences on skin barrier function and repair mechanisms. Dermatologic Therapy, 33(5), e13847.

Wilke, K., Martin, A., Terstegen, L., & Biel, S. S. (2007). A short history of sweat gland biology. International Journal of Cosmetic Science, 29(3), 169–179.

INDEX